THE ART OF
SMILE DESIGN

MARK K. NGUYEN, DDS

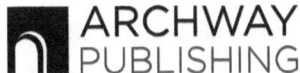

ARCHWAY
PUBLISHING

Archway Publishing books may be ordered through booksellers or by contacting:

Archway Publishing
1663 Liberty Drive
Bloomington, IN 47403
www.archwaypublishing.com
1 (888) 242-5904

ISBN: 978-1-4808-6594-5 (sc)
ISBN: 978-1-4808-6595-2 (e)

Library of Congress Control Number: 2018908593

Print information available on the last page.

Archway Publishing rev. date: 9/18/2018

CONTENTS

INTRODUCTION: ABOUT THE AUTHOR

My name is Mark Nguyen and cosmetic dentistry is my passion. I love to help patients discover the smile they never knew they could have, and I'm constantly working to better myself and my skills in order to offer them the best possible cosmetic dentistry options. Even more than that, however, I strive to ensure my patients have the healthiest, brightest smiles possible. When you work with me, you can rest assured that you're receiving great dental care on all fronts.

As will be reviewed in this book, it is important to choose a cosmetic dentist that not only has the qualifications but the experience needed to treat your teeth. My education, skill, and experience are what really set me apart from other dentists.

Education & Professional Societies

I received my Doctorate of Dental Surgery from the New York University College of Dentistry, a world-renowned dental college that emphasizes excellence in practice. I completed a general practice residency in Loma Linda at the VA Hospital and continued on to complete a clinical concentration program focused on cosmetic dentistry.

I have also completed a number of didactic and clinical training programs, including a 300-hour program on the placement of surgical implants and restoration and a 300-hour program encompassing cosmetic dentistry. In 2004, I completed a ten-week course for Invisalign certification that helped me gain an intimate understanding of the process and how it can help my patients. Additionally, I have been an Invisalign Premier Provider since 2016 – a designation only 5% of dentists enjoy.

I am incredibly proud of my education and the knowledge it has given me, and I'm happy to use that knowledge to help improve the lives of my patients. I also belong to a number of professional societies, including the:

- Spear Study Club
- California Dental Association
- American Dental Association
- American Academy of Implant Dentistry
- American Academy of Cosmetic Dentistry
- Academy of General Dentistry

Finally, I was named the Top Cosmetic Dentist by my board-certified colleagues in Orange Coast Magazine and featured by VoyageLA.

The bottom line? I work hard to ensure that your smile is healthy and looks the way you'd like it to. I'm qualified to do so and am confident in my ability to help you meet your goals. The goal of this book to help someone who doesn't have my education and experience understand how to get their smile to the best it can be and help them make informed decisions when choosing a dentist and procedure.

CHAPTER ONE

○ ○ ○ ○ ○ ○ ○◯◯◯ ◯ ◯◯◯◯○ ○ ○ ○ ○

Cosmetic Dentistry

A Brief History of Cosmetic Dentistry

When it comes to keeping your smile in optimal condition, the attention tends to be focused on maintaining oral health mostly through the avoidance or elimination of cavities and gingivitis. While this is certainly an understandable position, it is equally true that there tends to be relatively little focus upon the appearance of smiles and the assurance that teeth look as good as they feel. This is where the field of cosmetic dentistry comes in.

Cosmetic dentistry has made great strides over the past few decades. That is not to say, however, that it is an entirely new dental field. The desire to obtain a beautiful smile is not a modern one, and there are hints of what we now call cosmetic dentistry dating back as early as 700 B.C. During this time, bone and ivory dentures were created by the Etruscans, a wealthy civilization in ancient Italy. This indicates that individuals in this society valued a smile free of gaps and sought to create rudimentary dentures in order to help attain this vision of oral health and beauty.

There are numerous examples similar to the Etruscans dental practices. Creating dentures from bone, both human and animal, persisted until the 1800s. Ancient civilizations were also

1

known to practice teeth whitening, another common cosmetic dentistry procedure. The ancient Egyptians, for example, created a toothpaste composed of vinegar and pumice stone to help scrub away stains that developed upon their teeth. Early Romans also created a toothpaste that was designed to whiten teeth. Theirs contained urine as ammonia happens to be a natural method of tooth-whitening. Today, of course, there are far more pleasant and effective methods of tooth-whitening—but still, the desire for a bright smile is one that has persisted for centuries.

I say all of the above to communicate that cosmetic dentistry is an important dental field that has developed over the course of hundreds of years. It gained traction in the 1980s with the creation of more advanced dental care technology and has continued to improve in terms of both effectivity and popularity. Today, cosmetic dentistry aims to help patients achieve the perfect smile. Through the use of advanced restoration techniques as well as cosmetic procedures that promote both oral health and an attractive smile, this can be done.

Cosmetic Dentistry Today

As touched upon Cosmetic dentistry, as a field focused upon enhancing or restoring your smile, can involve a variety of procedures. This includes but is not limited to fixing chipped or broken teeth and purely cosmetic procedures, like applying dental veneers designed to help even out the appearance of your teeth. For patients hoping to improve and maintain their smiles, cosmetic dentistry is the best option.

It is important to note that cosmetic dentistry is more of an art than anything else. Because of this, it is imperative to seek out dentists specializing in this particular dental field when weighing options and potential solutions for your smile. Dentists who are not specially trained in cosmetic dentistry may not have the understanding and expertise needed to craft the perfect smile for you. Would you go to a doctor specializing in sinus health when what you really want is to change the appearance of your nose?

Hopefully, the answer to that is an emphatic no! Instead, you are more likely to opt for a surgeon who has experience in both enhancing and changing the appearance of a nose while maintaining its health and structure. This is the kind of service that a cosmetic dentist offers. Cosmetic dentists have the tools and knowledge needed to help create a smile you love while using methods that will work for your oral health and your budget.

Through using a wide array of tools and procedures, cosmetic dentists help every patient find his or her optimal smile. Some of these, like Invisalign Clear Braces, are incredibly easy and painless options which allow patients to make a big difference in the appearance of their smile without undergoing lengthy procedures or disrupting their lives in the process. Other procedures, like dental implants, can be a bit more involved and straddle the line between more traditional dentistry and cosmetic dentistry.

One thing to keep in mind is that dentists who focus on cosmetic procedures are just as qualified as "traditional" dentists when it comes to keeping your oral health in great shape. In fact, most cosmetic dentists have completed additional education to help keep them up-to-date with the latest options to ensure that their patients can smile with confidence due to the good health and appearance of their teeth. I am incredibly proud of my education and the skills it has given me. I received my doctorate of dental surgery from the New York University College of Dentistry, a world-renowned dental college that emphasizes excellence in practice. I also completed a general practice residency at the VA Hospital in Loma Linda and continued on to complete a clinical concentration program focused on cosmetic dentistry. Because of this, I am confident that my education and continued practice allows me to meet all the needs of my patients.

Is Cosmetic Dentistry Right for You?

Cosmetic dentistry is the best choice for anyone who needs or wants to have their smile restored or enhanced. The patient's motive for choosing a cosmetic dentistry procedure does not factor into their ability to obtain one. Whether you have teeth that have been damaged in an accident, lost due to poor oral health, or could simply be straighter or whiter, cosmetic dentistry exists to help you attain the best smile possible.

Something that is not often associated with dental work is self-confidence. Some individuals have perfectly healthy teeth, but they are unhappy with the appearance of their smile nonetheless. This is where cosmetic dentistry comes in. A cosmetic dentist can help maintain your oral health while also ensuring that you are happy with your smile. They can help even out gaps in teeth, create dentures or implants to replace lost teeth, and improve the shape, size, and color of your existing teeth. There are cosmetic options to help suit all needs! From fixing a small chip in a single tooth to revamping your entire smile, cosmetic dentistry has the tools to help you improve your self-confidence and live a happier life.

To clarify, someone with perfectly healthy teeth might seek out a cosmetic dentist to help create a more beautiful smile. Someone with discolored, misshapen, or missing teeth due to dental procedures or accidents might also seek out a cosmetic dentist. The reason behind your dissatisfaction with your teeth is something that will certainly be taken into consideration by a dentist experienced in cosmetic procedures, but it likely won't rule out your ability to acquire dental services.

Anyone who wants to work on his or her smile needs cosmetic dentistry. The great thing about this kind of dentistry is that, typically, the procedures are not overly invasive. That means that you can obtain a new smile without disrupting your daily life in a major way. If you're interested in improving your smile, don't hesitate to reach out! Cosmetic dentistry is a judgment-free zone where the only goal is to improve your oral health and leave you with a smile that is perfect in your eyes.

Does Cosmetic Dentistry Promote Oral Health?

There tends to be the misconception that cosmetic dentistry isn't concerned with oral health. Because cosmetic dentists have spent their time exploring the different procedures and tools that can be used in order to enhance their patients' smiles, some individuals conclude that appearance is all they focus on. And while this is an understandable conclusion, it is not a correct one.

Good oral health is a vital aspect of cosmetic dentistry. Without it, all of the work spent on improving an individual's smile could be lost when he or she needs a procedure caused by poor oral health. Good oral health is something that cannot be overstated.

Remember that you only get one set of teeth in your adulthood. If you don't take care of them, you could find yourself unable to pursue many things that you take for granted today. For example, the ability to properly chew, swallow, and enjoy your food becomes significantly harder once you start losing teeth. This is also true of things like speaking and smiling. Make no mistake: your teeth contribute greatly to your quality of life. Without them, everyday life looks very different.

Cosmetic dentists understand how important your oral health is to both your life and your satisfaction with your smile. That's one of the reasons why they take so much care to ensure that your smile is a healthy one. Once your teeth are in good shape, they can be considered a blank canvas upon which an experienced cosmetic dentist can create the smile of your dreams. It all begins with good oral health!

How Can Cosmetic Dentistry Help me?

Many people know about cosmetic dentistry in theory, but they aren't sure if they really need to pursue it. After all, can cosmetic procedures really have a significant impact on your life?

The answer, of course, is a resounding yes! To understand why it is first important to understand just how many different procedures fall under the umbrella of the cosmetic dentistry field. Some of them include:

- Invisalign Clear Braces
- Veneers
- Dental Implants
- Teeth Whitening
- Dental Bonding

The great thing about cosmetic dentistry is that it encompasses solutions for almost every issue out there. For example, let's say that you end up in an accident, and your teeth are injured in the process. While dentists are able to save the vast majority of them, unfortunately you end up losing two teeth as a result. And, of course, both of those teeth were in the front of your mouth. Now not only do you have trouble eating and chewing properly, but you also find it difficult to smile due to your altered appearance.

A cosmetic dentist can help! Dental implants are a great option in this situation. In chapter three dental implants will be discussed in more depth, but a brief overview is that they are "false teeth" implanted into your gums. In fact, many of them go right into the socket left behind by by your former tooth. The top of these implants are crowns, which look and function like a natural tooth.

Cosmetic dentists are skilled in the creation of these crowns. They can design implant crowns that will look like your true smile and, ultimately, enable you to eat and chew again properly.

Perhaps you didn't experience anything like the above, but simply don't like the way your teeth look. Many people find their teeth to be uneven in appearance and avoid smiling as a result. Well, a cosmetic dentist can help here, too! Cosmetic dentists have a plethora of tools at their disposal to help correct this issue, and they will pick the one that works best for your needs. Perhaps a set of veneers is in order? If that's not an option, dental bonding is a less-expensive alternative that dentists can use to create the appearance of even, cohesive teeth.

For individuals who find themselves struggling with their smile for a number of reasons, including the example above, there is a treatment available. Any number of issues can render a person unable to smile and speak easily because of the embarrassment that their teeth caused them. It might not seem like it, but this is a huge issue that can really impact the quality of your everyday life.

Think about the last time you watched something you found really amusing and laughed out loud with your family or friends. Were you plagued by concern over the appearance of your teeth, or were you able to smile naturally and unconsciously? For some people, the former is true. And these people often end up refusing to laugh or smile in public – and sometimes even in private – entirely. Their self-esteem takes a huge hit, but so does their mood and outlook on life.

If you never smile and are afraid to do so, your general mood could become less-than-optimistic. You might even find yourself depressed or chronically stressed, both of which can cause serious health issues. It might seem inconceivable that the appearance of your smile could impact your life so completely, but for some, it can have a significant negative effect.

The field of Cosmetic dentistry is designed specifically to help patients find the smile that they want. Cosmetic dentists work with their patients to not only ensure good oral health but to correct the appearance of their teeth. Whether this means installing dental implants or simply whitening teeth, the result is often the same: patients who were once painfully self-conscious about their smiles receive a "new lease on life" and achieve the smile of their dreams.

If you are dissatisfied with your smile, a cosmetic dentist like myself can help correct the appearance of your teeth and enhance your natural beauty.

CHAPTER TWO

o o o o o o o OOOO O OOOO o o o o o

Why a Beautiful Smile?

In the first chapter, we talked about why cosmetic dentistry is important and how it can help you achieve a beautiful smile. But you might be left wondering what exactly constitutes a beautiful smile and why you need one. This chapter is designed to help answer those questions! Let's take a look at what a beautiful smile looks like and how its presence can impact your life.

Benefits of a Beautiful Smile

A beautiful smile is one of your greatest attributes. Smiling at someone tends to cause the chain reaction of them smiling back. This, in turn, helps promote a positive image of yourself while also inspiring trust in the other person. A beautiful smile also increases your appeal and helps you seem more trustworthy. In other words, a beautiful smile can significantly help make your daily life easy as well as help you feel good about yourself and the world in which you live.

Many people believe that a beautiful smile is an entirely subjective opinion – that there are no universal rules that govern what makes a smile beautiful. This is not strictly true, however, as there are both objective attributes that define a beautiful smile as well as subjective opinions that can determine what an individual believes is a beautiful smile.

Because of the complexity behind what makes a beautiful smile, we will discuss both the objective and the subjective attributes that can allow a smile to be determined "beautiful" or not!

Why a Straight Smile is Healthiest

First, let's take a look at the objective attributes that create a beautiful smile, beginning with the characteristic of straight teeth. This is actually a rather important aspect of a beautiful smile for appearance and health reasons! To be blunt, straight teeth tend to be more aesthetically pleasing than teeth that are crooked – that means that most people will find a smile with straight teeth to be more beautiful than a smile with crooked teeth.

In addition, straight teeth are important for a host of other reasons. They enable individuals to floss and brush more easily and effectively which often relates directly to long-term oral health. This is especially important given that gum disease and tooth decay are both serious issues that can originate from poor oral hygiene and lead to serious health issues such as high blood sugar and heart disease.

Crooked, protruding, and crowded teeth are also problematic because they are more likely to break than straight teeth. This is perhaps even more dire for the athletically-inclined, as crooked teeth can be difficult to fit in mouth guards and can, ultimately, greatly diminish their effectivity. They can cause speech impediments that result in serious issues with self-confidence and negatively impact work or scholastic performance. Headaches are also side-effects of crooked and crowded teeth because of the increase in the amount of pressure on your jaw.

There are a variety of reasons why straight teeth make for a beautiful smile, and not all of them are purely aesthetic. A beautiful smile is a healthy smile, and crooked, protruding, and crowded teeth make it harder to achieve and maintain excellent dental health and cleanliness.

Discolored Smiles

The color of teeth is another characteristic to consider with regard to beautiful smiles. This one is fairly self-explanatory. Think about your favorite Hollywood actor or actress and picture their smile. Are their teeth yellow and discolored, or are they bright white? Chances are that their teeth are straight and almost blindingly white.

Teeth with little-to-no discoloration are an important part of a beautiful smile. They tend to be perceived as healthier than teeth that are heavily discolored, and can help a person appear more attractive and younger than they would otherwise appear.

Good health tends to be more attractive than poor health, and that standard holds true for teeth as well. Stained teeth or teeth that are discolored from medical procedures do not make for a beautiful smile.

Teeth Alignment

The third characteristic to look at is the alignment and evenness of teeth. A beautiful smile will have teeth that are, in addition to the above, even in alignment and spacing. That means that gaps are minimal and there are no missing teeth visible. Broken and chipped teeth go hand-in-hand with this characteristic as they greatly impact the overall uniform appearance of a smile.

Broken and chipped teeth are unattractive for a number of reasons. One of the main issues is that they make the smile in question seem uncared for and even weak, which can dramatically decrease the attractiveness of a smile. Chips and cracks also take away from the symmetry of an individual's smile and face.

As shown, several objective aspects contribute to a beautiful smile. That means that these characteristics are almost universally agreed upon as qualities that constitute a beautiful smile by dentists and patients alike. With that being said, there is a great deal of subjectivity to what is and what is not considered a beautiful smile, which we will review in the next section.

Subjective Characteristics of a Beautiful Smile

As the old saying goes, "beauty is in the eye of the beholder". That is certainly true when it comes to smiles. Almost everyone has specific things that make or break a smile in their minds, which is why employing the help of an experienced cosmetic dentist skilled at combining personal preference with objective beautiful smile characteristics is so important.

One subjective characteristic of a beautiful smile is the size. Some people prefer a large, wide smile full of bright white teeth while others would rather see more demure smiles. Some individuals are particularly taken with smiles that show a lot of gum, which is a preference that goes against the conventional wisdom that states only a small amount of your gums should be visible.

Some people prefer a smile in which every last tooth is uniform and even. This is a look that is often accomplished through the use of porcelain veneers, which help create a natural-looking and even smile. Others, of course, prefer a more "natural" appearance and like to see some variety in their smiles.

At this point, you might be wondering why, exactly, this is an important discussion. I think it's necessary to highlight that every patient has a specific smile in mind, and it might not be a smile that is conventionally perfect in its appearance. The characteristics of beautiful smiles can be quite subjective, and often require a cosmetic dentist to carefully weave together a patient's opinions regarding their smile together with some of the more objective aspects of attractive smiles.

In other words, it is okay if your smile doesn't perfectly adhere to the objective characteristics discussed above. You can have a beautiful smile without meeting all of them. The most important thing is that you find your smile attractive and are happy with it. An experienced cosmetic dentist, like myself, will be able to help you achieve the smile of your dreams. You can have a beautiful smile, no matter what your teeth look like today (or what you want your teeth to look like). As long as they are healthy and strong, beautiful smiles can differ greatly from person to person.

Does your smile really impact your appearance?

Teeth are often taken for granted in many areas of life, and appearance is no exception. Many people roll their eyes at the thought of investing in their smile and believe that their teeth don't impact their lives or other people's perception of them in any way. This is, of course, not the case. While we try not to judge by looks alone, in reality, that's often exactly how we form opinions of others. Sometimes this is even unconscious in nature.

People with beautiful smiles project a more positive image than those without. A recent study conducted by Kelton Research investigated this idea. Their conclusions were quite definitive in nature. The study, which surveyed over 1,000 American citizens, explored how a person's smile impacts other's impression of them. It found that beautiful smiles – smiles with white, straight, and uniform teeth – were associated with wealth, success, and trustworthiness by participants. In contrast, crooked and uneven teeth were associated with the exact opposite.

Additionally, people with beautiful smiles were perceived as being far more attractive than individuals with problematic smiles (stained, cracked, or broken teeth) even when the rest of the features in question were similar.

According to the study, the condition of your smile is tied to your character and trustworthiness. If your smile is healthy and straight, you have an advantage when it comes to things like job interviews. Even beyond that, however, is the fact that participants indicated that individuals with beautiful smiles were more "dateable" and "worthy" of getting to know. Your smile impacts how you are perceived by the rest of the world as well as what kind of people are willing to speak with you and get to know you.

This doesn't mean that you can't make a good impression with problematic teeth, of course, but it does show that individuals with beautiful and healthy teeth have an easier time doing so. Your teeth are a standout feature and should be well-cared-for. And yes, your teeth have a huge impact on your appearance. In addition to the disadvantages mentioned before, stained and crooked teeth can make you look older than you really are. Bright white and straight teeth, on the other hand, make you seem much younger

Is it possible to obtain a beautiful smile even if you have less-than-perfect teeth?

Absolutely! This is a question that I hear all of the time, and I cannot emphasize this enough: you can achieve the smile of your dreams with the right cosmetic dentist. That's true even if your teeth are not in ideal shape. Your dentist can work with you to improve the health of your teeth while also ensuring that their appearance is exactly what you were hoping to see. In fact, it only makes sense that if you have less-than-perfect teeth, you'd see the services of an experienced cosmetic dentist, right? If your teeth were perfect, there wouldn't be anything to fix!

Something else to keep in mind is the fact that cosmetic dentistry can be something as simple as an hour-long whitening session. People tend to envision complex, expensive procedures when they think about cosmetic dentistry, but that couldn't be farther from the truth. The process that your dentist takes will depend upon what, exactly, you'd like your teeth to look like. For many people, a whitening session is a huge change and gives them a smile they love.

Even if you have crooked and discolored teeth but would like to have a beautiful smile, don't worry – there are options to help you achieve the smile of your dreams, too! Options like Invisalign Clear Braces can sometimes be used to correct and straighten your teeth painlessly and effortlessly over the course of several weeks. Once your teeth are straighter, you might look into cosmetic options like whitening procedures or porcelain veneers.

Don't stay away from a cosmetic dentist because you don't think they can help. I've personally seen all sorts of smiles in my career, and it's possible to help individuals in almost any situation achieve a brighter, healthier, and happier smile. You have nothing to lose by speaking with a cosmetic dentist for more information, so I urge you to take that first step and see what we can do to help you love your smile.

Can anyone have a beautiful smile?

In short, the answer to this question is yes! It is never too late to invest in a smile that you absolutely love. There are tooth restoration options for just about every problem you can imagine, and many of them are probably faster and simpler than you might think. Even if you are suffering from missing teeth, there are procedures available to help not only improve the appearance of your smile but to also restore function and enable you to speak clearly or chew properly again.

One thing to keep in mind is that if your teeth are still developing, it might be wise to wait on certain cosmetic procedures until that process has completed. That doesn't mean that there isn't a cosmetic dentistry solution for your needs, but rather that some of the more complex restoration procedures are designed to be performed on mature teeth.

No matter how your current smile looks, you can achieve a beautiful smile with the help of cosmetic dentistry. Again, do not hesitate simply because you don't believe your teeth are in good shape. Even if they aren't, fixing the problems and attaining better oral health is within reach! Cosmetic procedures can be applied once your teeth are healthy and strong.

Whether you are young or old, a beautiful smile is within your grasp. All you need is a knowledgeable cosmetic dentist to help determine and discuss with you the best procedures for your needs. You might be surprised at just how advanced modern dentistry really is.

As a final note, I want to take a moment to reiterate just how important your smile can be for both your physical and mental well-being as well as your appearance. If you are not happy with your smile and find it difficult to smile or even speak in public, your self-confidence will take a significant hit. Your overall perspective will also decrease, and you might even end up struggling with depression or shame.

In addition to how your smile impacts your health and appearance, it also impacts how others perceive you. If you want to be seen as a capable and successful individual, then you might find it worthwhile to invest in your smile and cultivate the very best appearance possible.

Instead of worrying about your smile, why not do something about it? Modern cosmetic dentistry can help you achieve the smile of your dreams. If you want a beautiful smile, all you have to do is reach out to an experienced cosmetic dentist!

CHAPTER THREE

How to Attain a Beautiful Smile

For some, the idea of obtaining a beautiful smile might seem something like a pipe dream. This is especially true if your smile is significantly "flawed" – if it has a variety of imperfections that are noticeable. It is important to me that you understand that this doesn't have to be the case. Cosmetic dentistry can give you the smile you've always wanted.

As an experienced cosmetic dentist, I've seen it all. Almost every problem or issue you can imagine might affect a smile is one that I am already familiar with. And by working through those problems systematically, I am able to give my patients the aesthetic that they are hoping. It's not impossible, no matter how your smile currently looks. Thanks to the advancements in modern cosmetic dentistry, even the most damaged or misshapen of smiles can achieve perfection.

I understand how hard it can be to envision a beautiful smile. For many patients, the road to that end goal often seems like a very long one. That doesn't have to be the case. And, even if you need to have multiple procedures completed to help make your smile the healthiest and straightest possible, this is something that we can work on consistently. An experienced doctor, like myself, will work with you to find the best schedule and timeline for your smile enhancement process.

So, what kind of procedures might you face if you choose to correct the imperfections plaguing your smile and gain a bright, beautiful set of teeth? As briefly discussed earlier, there is truly a wide array of tools available to the cosmetic dentist. For every problem and almost every budget, there is a procedure that can be done to help improve a smile.

Because of the multitude of procedures available, it is important to understand how and why each one might be beneficial for your smile. This next section will have more in-depth descriptions of each procedure, including how invasive it is and what the recovery time might look like. It is very important to be well-informed before choosing any cosmetic dental option, and a deep understanding of what happens during these procedures might make undergoing them a bit less intimidating to think about.

Common Cosmetic Dental Procedures

If you are interested in perfecting your smile, there are a few procedures that are more common than others. This does not mean that you will have to experience all – or even one – of the below options. This is meant to serve as a reference, nothing more. With that in mind, let's get started!

Invisalign Clear Braces

You are probably familiar with orthodontic metal braces. They are a dental device attached to teeth and connected by wires in order to help straighten them. This is usually something that is done during adolescence, however metal braces are also an option for adults. The popularity of this particular procedure, however, wanes due to a number of factors, including:

- The amount of time it takes to apply and remove the braces.
- The way in which traditional metal braces dictate what can and cannot be eaten.
- The difficulty of maintaining traditional metal braces.
- The discomfort that comes along with the metal wire adjustment.

This is not to say that metal braces no longer have a place in dentistry, of course, but rather that there are better options available for many patients.

Instead of investing in traditional metal braces, Invisalign Clear Braces are a much simpler and more pleasant alternative. These aligners are designed to reposition your teeth and help straighten your smile over a period of time. Choosing Invisalign Clear Braces are an improvement over traditional braces in a number of different ways.

As opposed to sitting in a dentist's chair for hours while braces are applied, Invisalign Clear Braces are easy to snap on and off of your teeth. As a patient, you would go through a fitting process where a 3D scan is taken of your mouth and teeth that is then sent to a specialized lab. Your aligners are custom-created for your needs and sent back to your dentist's office. After a final fitting, leave with your clear aligners! All in all, the process is incredibly quick and easy.

Invisalign Clear Braces do not limit what you can and cannot eat. Because the aligners can be easily removed and inserted over your teeth, you can easily eat the food you want – even if it's something small or sticky – by removing the aligner. Once you are finished eating, all you need to do is brush your teeth and pop the aligners right back in place. In other words, you don't have to spend hours carefully flossing rotten bits of food from between wires, which is the unenviable fate of individuals opting for traditional metal braces.

Traditional metal braces can be difficult to keep clean. Eating something particularly sticky will result in stubborn residue stuck all over them, which means that you have to spend ages carefully cleaning them every night. Additionally, food often gets stuck between traditional metal braces and your teeth, leading to an arduous routine of extensive flossing every day. Alternatively, Invisalign Clear Braces are easy to clean and disinfect. You also don't have to worry about wires bending or breaking, another common issue that individuals with traditional braces experience.

Finally, it is important to talk about just how comfortable Invisalign Clear Braces are. Traditional braces are affixed to your teeth and are periodically tightened to help pull your teeth into position. This can be a painful process for the patient, and result in sensitive teeth as well as significant jaw pain and headaches. Invisalign Clear Braces, on the other hand, are designed to be carefree and comfortable. You are generally given a set of clear aligners that are swapped out weekly or every few weeks. This very gently guides your teeth into place over a period of time, gradually improving your smile without extra work or pain.

The best part about Invisalign Clear Braces? Well, it's right there in the name: they're clear! You can wear Invisalign Clear Braces without anyone being the wiser. This discretion is not possible for individuals with traditional metal braces.

Invisalign is a great option for almost anyone, but especially for adults who don't want to broadcast their dental habits to the world. You can wear these clear braces to work, on dates, and even around friends and family without attracting extra attention to your teeth. They allow you to straighten your smile on your own terms, on your own time.

Porcelain Veneers

Another commonly utilized – and extremely effective – cosmetic procedure is the application of porcelain veneers. It can be difficult for people to wrap their heads around the option of veneers, because the thought of affixing something to the outside of your teeth might not sound like a pleasant experience. It is understandable to be hesitant when choosing this procedure. It is my hope that with a better understanding of how this cosmetic option works, you will be able to make a more informed decision about the best treatment for your teeth.

Porcelain veneers are a safe and incredibly effective way to transform your smile. It is essential to note that your original teeth are not harmed in the process! While they might undergo a bit of shaping, your teeth will remain just as healthy as they were before the procedure. And if you want dramatic results that give you an even, bright, and straight smile – a "perfect" smile, if you will – then porcelain veneers are a great way to go.

Porcelain veneers are very thin pieces of porcelain that are placed over your teeth. Think of a crown and you have the basic idea. These porcelain caps are carefully crafted to look natural and beautiful and are bonded into place one by one. You won't even be able to feel the difference between the way your natural teeth and your porcelain veneers feel!

So, how exactly are porcelain veneers applied and prepared? First, your cosmetic dentist will take accurate molds or a 3D scan of your teeth and mouth to ensure that the veneers that will be attached will fit your teeth perfectly. They are custom-created to fit both your current teeth as well as the overall look you are hoping to achieve through their application.

By your second appointment, the veneers – created from the molds of your teeth – will be ready at your dentist's office. Your teeth will most likely be contoured a bit to make sure that porcelain adheres to them well, and then the veneers are bonded into place (after checking to make sure that your bite is accurate, of course). Just like that, you have a brand-new smile!

With proper care and maintenance, your veneers should last you for many years to come. While they are thin, they are also incredibly strong once bonded to your teeth. With that said, they can pick up stains if they are not cared for – just like your natural teeth – so it is important to practice good oral maintenance.

Dental Implants

So far, we've been talking about how to alter your existing teeth to create a great smile. In some instances, however, one of the biggest challenges you face when it comes to transforming your smile is a lack of teeth. While dentists tend to do everything possible to save natural teeth, there are circumstances where this is simply not possible. If your teeth have been damaged beyond repair, for example, or become diseased or infected, you might end up needing to have them pulled.

Before we talk about dental implants specifically, let's take a minute to talk about why maintaining a full set of teeth is important. You might think of your teeth as permanent fixtures in your mouth – structures that are firmly in place and do not move without quite a bit of encouragement. In reality, your teeth remain in place mostly because of the pressure of your other teeth. Together, your teeth fit together to form a strong and cohesive whole, in other words. But if you remove one or more of them, the remaining teeth suddenly have a lot more room to explore.

After having teeth removed, it is common for patients to see their other teeth begin drifting out of place. This is bad for several reasons. First of all, drifting (and missing) teeth impact your bite. A change in your bite can have a variety of undesirable consequences, including increasing the pressure on certain teeth and ultimately damaging them as a result. Drifting teeth also impact both your smile and the structural integrity of your mouth. It is important, then, to replace missing teeth as quickly as possible.

When looking for a tooth restoration option that will help return your smile to its natural glory, dental implants are one of the best options out there. It is best to think of a dental implant as two separate entities. There is a metal post that is inserted into your jaw, and there is the crown that is placed over the post to complete your smile. Whenever possible, the post is placed in the same place where your missing tooth once resided. Eventually, it will bond with your jaw and will be just as functional as a natural tooth.

In regards to cosmetic dentistry, the more interesting part of a dental implant might be the crown. A dental crown, often created from porcelain or ceramic, is carefully sculpted to match the rest of your teeth. It is then placed over the post of the implant. Dental implants tend to look extremely natural and, even better, function as natural teeth do once they have healed.

It is important to note that the dental implant installation procedure is a more invasive one that some of the other procedures available. It is a surgical procedure that requires the services of an experienced oral surgeon or cosmetic dentist and can take several hours to complete. After the post is installed into your mouth, the healing process can take anywhere from four to eight or so weeks. You will need to visit your dentist during this time so that they can monitor your implant and ensure that it is healing properly.

Many patients liken the healing process of dental implant surgery to that of having a wisdom tooth removed. It is not necessarily a pleasant experience, in other words, but it is also not exceedingly painful or complicated. And once your implant has healed and your crown is in place, you will have a beautiful and functional smile that should last the rest of your life – with proper care and maintenance!

Teeth Whitening

People tend to think that all cosmetic dentistry is invasive, but that couldn't be further from the truth! In fact, sometimes all you need is a quick teeth whitening session to completely transform your smile and see the results you're hoping for. Many of my patients are shocked at just how much a professional teeth whitening session can impact the way that they look.

Teeth become discolored over time – this is normal. This is something that happens to everyone in varying degrees. The amount of tooth discoloration – and, therefore, the number of teeth whitening sessions needed to remove the stains – depends heavily upon the foods you eat and the things you drink. There are certain foods and beverages that can really wreak havoc upon the appearance of your teeth. Some that can darken the appearance of your smile include:

- Tea
- Coffee
- Soda
- Citrus
- Red Wine
- White Wine
- Sweets
- Pomegranate
- Blueberries
- Blackberries
- Acidic Food

Avoiding or limiting the amount of food and drinks listed above you consume will help limit the amount of discoloration and stains that your teeth pick up. You might also want to keep in mind that there are certain foods and drinks that can help keep your teeth bright and white:

- Cheese
- Water
- Strawberries

- Nuts
- Fruit Rich in Fiber

Why are we talking about the food and drinks that keep your teeth bright and the ones that don't? Because teeth whitening doesn't last forever. If you have your teeth whitened and then go right back to drinking multiple cups of coffee and dark soda a day, for example, the whitening effects are less likely to stay prominent for any length of time. It is important that you understand how teeth whitening works before you invest in it, and that you take the time to think about your diet and how you can alter it to ensure that your newly brightened teeth stay white as long as possible.

As far as the procedure itself, it's an easy one! There are a few different ways to go, but most dentists will have a UV light whitening system that will be focused upon your teeth for an hour or so, during which time your teeth could lighten quite a few shades. Depending on the severity of the stains and discoloration, you might need multiple sessions to achieve the results you want, but the process is an easy and non-invasive one.

Dental Bonding

We've already talked about porcelain veneers and how they can be applied to create a uniform and beautiful smile. If you aren't interested in veneers or they are out of reach, however, don't panic – your quest for the perfect smile is not yet over! Another option to keep in mind is that of dental bonding.

Like porcelain veneers, dental bonding is the process of adding material to your teeth in order to create a cohesive and more perfect smile. Unlike porcelain veneers, the material is not placed completely over your teeth to create an entirely different smile. Instead, it is applied to specific areas of a tooth that are perhaps cracked or uneven. The composite resin is moldable at first, which leaves your dentist plenty of time to shape it to perfectly match your teeth.

Once the right shape has been acquired, the resin is permanently bonded to your teeth. This material can even be dyed to match the color of the rest of your teeth, however, it is a good idea to reach out to an experienced and knowledgeable cosmetic dentist such as myself in order to ensure that the results appear natural. Remember that the person applying this resin must be able to sculpt even minute details in order to make sure that the results are flawless, so a skilled cosmetic dentist is the best person to turn to for this procedure.

Dental bonding is a good option for individuals who do not want veneers. While the resin is not meant to completely cover your teeth (and therefore transform it completely) it can work well to correct issues like chipped or uneven teeth that detract from the overall appearance of your smile. It is a great solution for small problems that don't warrant veneers, but it is probably not the best solution if the issues you are attempting to address are numerous and prominent.

CHAPTER FOUR

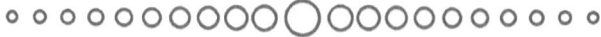

Celebrity Smiles and their Uniqueness

Because celebrities often have the smiles most hope to achieve, it can be helpful to take a look at various celebrities and their famous smile. Most celebrity smiles are considered to be perfect, yet are all very unique, which is another example of the objective and subjective characteristics that might make up a beautiful smile.

Many of my patients come into my office with the hopes of emulating the smile of a certain celebrity, and I find that it's sometimes helpful to use their teeth as examples when discussing what makes a smile beautiful. Because a beautiful smile is one that adheres to certain objectives as well as subjective standards, these specific examples help me give the patient the smile they desire most. Your smile is, speaking frankly, one of your greatest assets! Teeth that are straight, proportional, and bright white are universally seen as attractive. These are three factors that objectively help determine whether a smile is "beautiful".

With that said, don't discount the subjectivity involved in determining beauty. In fact, there are many examples of individuals who don't have a picture-perfect smile who, nonetheless, possess a pleasing appearance, highlighting the subjectivity to beautiful smiles. This is true even in Hollywood, an industry famously focused on the importance of youth and idealistic attractiveness. While some movie stars do boast a beautiful smile, others have smiles whose little "quirks" help increase their appeal.

In other words, beautiful smiles don't always equal "perfect" smiles. Instead, they are perfect for the individual wearing them. That's an important distinction to keep in mind when you're looking to enhance your smile. You don't have to give up unique characteristics that you like simply because they aren't part of a conventionally perfect smile. It is more than possible to have a smile that is beautiful while not perfect, and skillful dental cosmetic procedures can help enhance your smile around the perceived imperfections. You just have to find an experienced dentist who understands the ins and outs of smile enhancement.

These ideas will be easier to understand with specific examples in mind. We'll look at celebrities with conventionally "perfect" and beautiful smiles as well as those with beautifully imperfect smiles.

Anne Hathaway

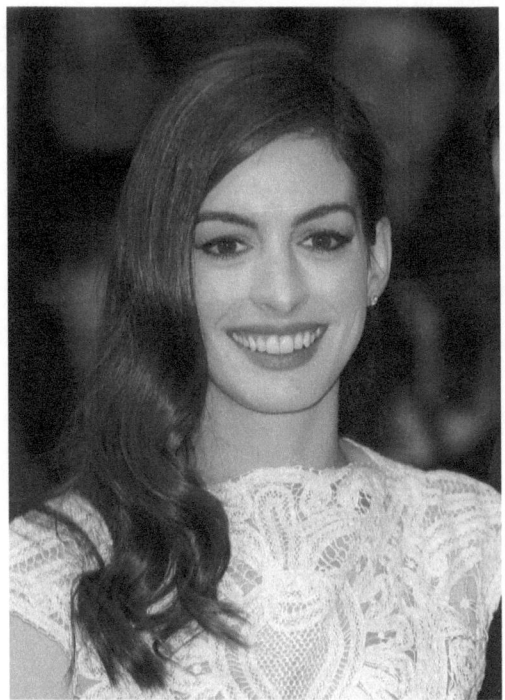

Figure 1 Featureflash Photo Agency//Shutterstock = Anne Hathaway

Anne Hathaway is probably one of the best examples of a celebrity with a conventionally perfect smile. There are a few different things that make her smile so distinctive and appealing. First of all, note that her teeth are straight and evenly spaced. Their alignment is just about perfect, and their appearance is uniform and cohesive. Her gum-to-teeth ratio – the amount of gum that shows when she smiles – is also perfect, placing the attention squarely upon her teeth and her smile rather than taking attention away from her beauty.

Hathaway's smile is one of the most emulated around. It is often possible to attain similar results using a few different methods depending upon the starting smile in question. Invisalign Clear Braces can be used to help straight teeth and cure misalignment or crowding issues. Teeth whitening treatments can help dull or discolored teeth recover their shine, and porcelain veneers can better shape and even out teeth to help achieve that picture-perfect smile.

Anna Paquin

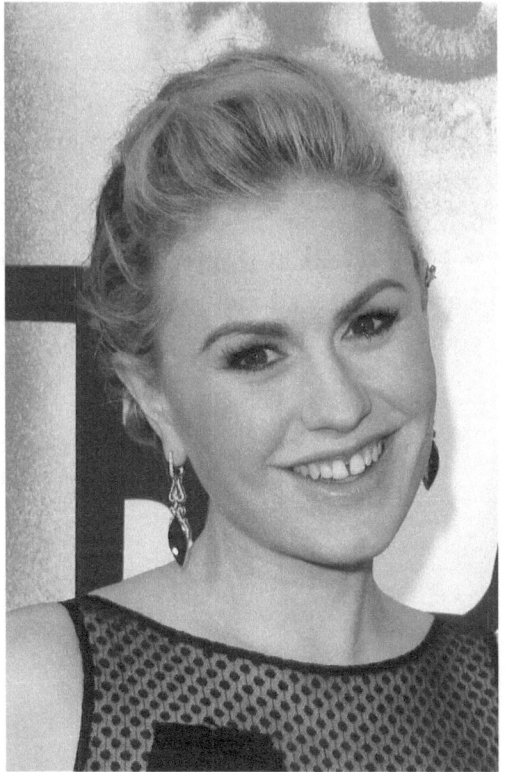

Figure 2 s_bukley//Shutterstock = Anna Paquin.

Perhaps best-known for her portrayal of Sookie Stackhouse on HBO's True Blood, Anna Paquin's smile is an immediately noteworthy one. In contrast to Anne Hathaway, it is not a "perfect" smile – at least not in the traditional sense. It is a memorable smile that has captivated many people, however, and it is noteworthy precisely because it is not perfect. Her teeth are not perfectly spaced, with the gap between her two front teeth lending them an endearing quality.

Paquin might not have the most perfect smile, but she has one of the most memorable in Hollywood. Her smile doesn't seem to have hurt her success, and her fans find it quite attractive and endearing despite its quirks. It is important to note, however, that while her smile isn't technically perfect, it also doesn't have any serious problems. There are no crowded, crooked, or discolored teeth, and, aside from her front teeth being slightly misaligned, her smile appears to be a healthy one that adheres to conventional ideas regarding what makes a smile beautiful.

If your goal is to fix your smile but have the quirks in your smile similar to Paquin's remain, that is possible. A skilled cosmetic dentist will be able to create a beautiful and healthy grin without losing any of your smile's uniqueness.

Tom Cruise

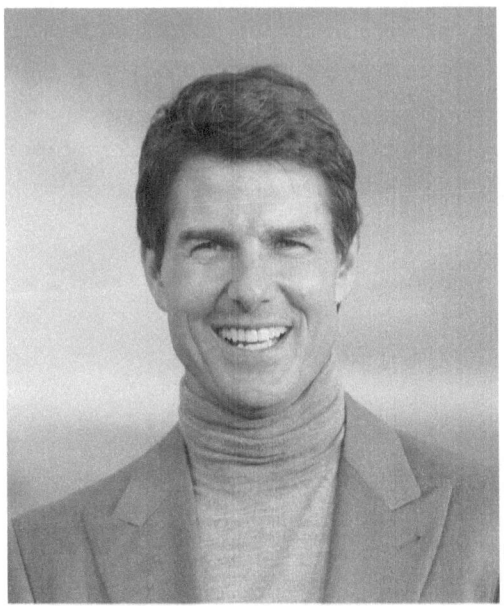

Figure 3 DFree//Shutterstock = Tom Cruise.

Tom Cruise has a great smile; one that is often referenced in the mainstream media and pop culture. It's bright and eye-catching – and imperfect, surprisingly enough. This is a fact that confounds many patients seeking to attain a dramatic smile like that of Cruise. Much like Paquin, Cruise has a smile that conforms to conventional ideas of dental health and beauty in many ways but it has its own flaws. You won't be able to "unsee" it after I point it out, either, so take a moment to savor the illusion a moment longer if you must!

Look at the picture above and focus on Cruises' teeth. Specifically, look at their alignment with the rest of his face. Do you see how he has one tooth squarely in the middle of his smile? Compare that with Hathaway's smile a few pages above. Her two front teeth are virtually perfectly placed in the middle of her mouth. Cruise, on the other hand, has a smile that is dominated by a "mono-tooth" – a tooth that is situated in the center of his face.

Despite the imperfection in Cruises' smile, his story is one of dental success! He's not alone, either, with other celebrities weighing in on their positive experiences with cosmetic dental treatment, too.

Cosmetic dentistry helped give a plethora of celebrities an attractive and healthy smile, even if it still contains small imperfections.

Zachary Levi

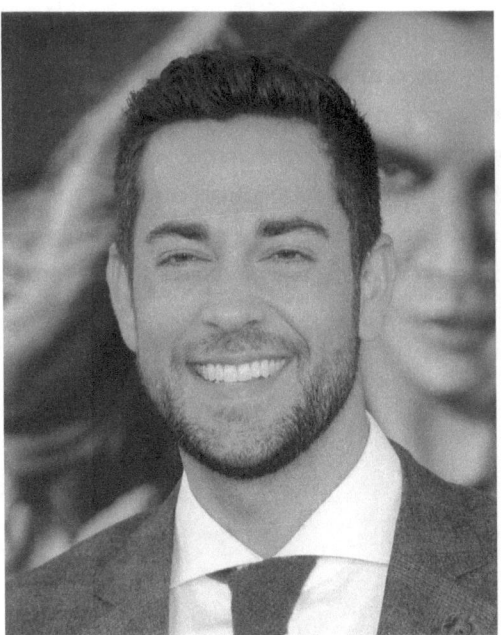

Figure 4 DFree//Shutterstock = Zachary Levi

Primarily known for his voice acting in games like Fallout: New Vegas as well as his work in TV series like Chuck, Heroes Reborn, and the movie Shazam!, Zachary Levi has the male counterpart to Hathaway's perfect smile. His teeth are straight and bright white. They are also well-spaced and are aligned well in proportion to the rest of his face. Like Hathaway, it is often possible to attain similar results using various cosmetic dentistry methods. These include things like teeth whitening, Invisalign Clear Braces, and porcelain veneers.

There's a Perfect Smile for Everyone

If you're looking for a perfect smile, you are in luck! The advancements made in cosmetic dentistry have made it possible to fix and perfect even the most imperfect of smiles. By consulting with a cosmetic dentist and discussing your goals for your smile, you can choose the right procedures and steps to achieving the smile of your dreams. Celebrities don't have to be the only ones with the perfect teeth, you too can have a smile ready to appear on the cover of a magazine.

∘ ∘ ∘ ∘ ∘ ∘ ○○○○○ ○ ○○○○○○ ∘ ∘ ∘ ∘

CHAPTER FIVE

Invisalign Clear Braces

The importance of a beautiful and healthy smile as well as the various ways to obtain one has now been thoroughly covered in the previous chapters. With that said, there is one option in particular that is often underutilized especially when considering the incredible results it offers patients. Invisalign Clear Braces are an incredible way to straighten teeth and enhance your smile while expending little effort along the way. It's an easy, effective, and affordable cosmetic dentistry option, and one that I think deserves a bit more discussion.

What is Invisalign?

In previous chapters Invisalign was briefly outlined as a potential option for patients, however, for those strongly considering the benefits of this procedure, I will go into more detail. The Invisalign Clear Braces system is a bit of a cross between cosmetic dentistry and orthodontia. To explain it clearly, this system is exactly what the name implies: a set of clear braces that are designed to easily and painlessly align and straighten your teeth. These aren't braces in the traditional sense they are not attached to teeth and tightened by wires like conventional braces. Instead, they are a set of clear trays that can be easily placed or removed.

The braces work to straighten and align teeth, and can be an effective tool in remedying the following issues:

- Gaps between your teeth
- Overcrowding in your mouth
- Basic bite issues and irregularities
- Teeth shifting after traditional braces are removed
- Crossbites
- Overbites

If you find yourself thinking about investing in teeth straightening options, consider speaking with a cosmetic dentist about Invisalign Clear Braces. You might be surprised at the dramatic results you can achieve with them, as well as just how easy the process can be. In case you're still not entirely sure what makes Invisalign a more attractive option to some patients over conventional braces, let's talk about the benefits the Invisalign Clear Braces treatment offers.

Advantages of Invisalign

One of the main downsides to conventional braces is the amount of time they must be worn paired with the discomfort they often caused. Because these braces can significantly affect the wearer's ability to easily eat and speak, wearing them for months on end can often prove to be quite a chore. Invisalign Clear Braces, on the other hand, cause patients little, if any, discomfort. That is because they are designed completely differently from conventional braces.

Traditional braces are attached to teeth permanently – they must be removed by an orthodontist, and they are firmly affixed in place from day one. Additionally, they have to be adjusted repeatedly throughout the course of the treatment process. This means that patients have to make repeated visits to their orthodontist to have the braces manually tightened, often leading to significant pain and discomfort.

With Invisalign, patients receive a set of clear braces pairs that are designed to fit over their teeth. They make small adjustments over time, with patients typically receiving a schedule that tells them when to switch to the next pair of braces in the kit. This is done incrementally so that the wearer feels minimal discomfort. Additionally, these clear aligners are easy to put over your teeth as well as to remove – all you have to do is slide them on and tug them off again when necessary. This is great for a variety of reasons, perhaps the most prominent of which is ease of eating.

With traditional braces, wearers must be careful with the kind of food they eat. Certain food, like gum, can stick to the braces and must be carefully cleaned. Additionally, it is not uncommon for food to get stuck under the braces themselves, leading to rotting food that must be painstakingly removed using various tools and methods. Invisalign Clear Braces, on the other hand, pose no such issues. You can even remove the clear aligners when it's time to eat so that you can keep both the braces and your teeth in great shape. You can brush your teeth after eating and clear away any food remnants as you normally would.

Finally, the appearance of Invisalign Clear Braces is something that deserves attention. Take a moment and think about traditional braces. Chances are good that you could immediately envision their appearance on teeth. That's because, in the past, they were extremely visible and noticeable. They created an impression upon the mind of individuals wearing them as well as those seeing them. Now, take a moment and think about Invisalign Clear Braces.

What came to mind? If you weren't sure what to think or simply saw a set of clear trays, you might already see where I'm going with this. Because they are, by design, clear, Invisalign Clear Braces don't attract any attention at all. They fit over your teeth and look natural, meaning that no one but you ever has to know that you're wearing them if you don't feel like sharing. Invisalign is a low-profile alternative to traditional braces that work towards the same goal.

To quickly sum up, Invisalign Clear Braces offer patients a wide variety of benefits when compared to conventional braces. This is true in design as well as practical function. If you are in need of teeth straightening and basic alignment help, it is a good idea to speak with an experienced cosmetic dentist about Invisalign Clear Braces as an alternative to traditional braces and how they can help improve your smile. Not only are they more convenient, but Invisalign is virtually pain-free and make maintaining your oral hygiene easy. They also won't impact your self-confidence or draw undue attention to your appearance.

The Invisalign Process

You might be wondering exactly how Invisalign works and what you can expect. The fact of the matter is that it's surprisingly simple! Let's take a look at how it happens at my clinic.

At the initial consult, you can expect to meet with the dentist who will be treating you. This is the perfect time to ask questions about the process and what treatment will be like. You will also have a 3D scan conducted to start the process and generate your specific treatment plan. The treatment coordinator is also an important part of this first consult, and you'll have the chance to meet with them and ask them any questions you might have about the suggested treatment. The coordinator will also cover financing options during this initial consult as well.

Once the treatment plan has been accepted, the 3D scans of your teeth will be sent to Invisalign to create your custom aligners. You'll come back to pick them up once they are ready, and at this point in time the cosmetic dentist overseeing your treatment will make sure that they fit properly and show you how to remove and insert them properly.

Typically, I have my patients switch their aligners every two weeks. With that said, we also offer Propel technology that can accelerate treatment time and potentially cut it in half. This is a great option if you have a specific date by which time you need your teeth to be straight and aligned. Brides hoping to look their best for their wedding photos, for example, often find this option to be particularly useful.

If you think Invisalign Clear Braces are the right option for your teeth, reach out to an experienced dentist today for more information about how they can help. I'm always happy to assist my patients in finding the very best treatment plan for their needs.

CHAPTER SIX

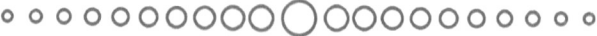

How to Choose a
Cosmetic Dentist

One thing that we haven't yet covered in this book is how exactly you can choose a cosmetic dentist. Should you just do a quick search on Google and pick the first result you see?

Well, of course not. If you needed to visit a specialist because your leg was fractured, would you just pick a random doctor and hope for the best? Most people, I wager, would say "no". We tend to do our research carefully when it comes to finding physicians to treat our bodies. We want the very best care possible – the doctor who is best equipped to treat our issue and help us bounce back to full health. With that goal in mind, people tend to be picky about their specialists. And, to be frank, that's good! It's always a good idea to arm yourself with knowledge when you're making a decision that could impact your health.

This same level of research and pickiness should be applied when choosing a cosmetic dentist as well. It is necessary to take the time to research your potential dentists and look into their experience and education. Many people are all too quick to accept whatever dentist happens to be close by. They opt for convenience rather than knowledge and expertise, and make the mistake of assuming that all dentists are created equal. Just as that specialist who can help heal your leg has specialized knowledge in their field, so, too, do dentists. What makes a dentist great in one area of dentistry might not help them out in another.

The best thing you can do for your smile when looking to enhance it is find the right dentist. It is my hope is that by giving you the knowledge and tools you need to narrow down your cosmetic dentist choice, you'll be able to find a dentist that excels in areas that are relevant to your goals and your needs.

Finding the Right Cosmetic Dentist is Important

Let's go back to the specialist example. When you fracture or break a bone, you will likely see an orthopedic doctor to determine the extent of the damage as well as the best way to go about healing it. That doctor is one that spent years of their lives studying the way that bones break and heal. They have specialized knowledge in this area that is not equaled by a general practitioner because the general practitioner didn't dedicate their time studying one specific area of healthcare. Instead, they focused on a more general scope in order to provide patients with great care when faced with a variety of more mundane issues.

Does that mean that the general practitioner isn't a good doctor? Of course not! They are likely invaluable to your health. What I'm trying to illustrate with this example is that these doctors have very different skill sets and fill different roles in healthcare. The orthopedic doctor will help you heal your broken bones and move on with your life – and out of their office. It is unlikely that you'll see that specialist again once you are fully healed and back to 100% health. You'll still see your general practitioner often, however, because they help keep you healthy on a day-to-day basis. One of these doctors is focused on a single area while the other is focused on a general sense of health.

The same can be said of dentists. Family dentists, for example, likely spent much of their education learning about the general dental needs of individuals of all ages. They're fantastic dentists who work hard to keep your teeth healthy. But when you need more specialized care, doesn't it make sense to seek out a specialized dentist?

Cosmetic dentists have spent years of their lives learning about cosmetic dentistry in addition to learning about general dental care. They have their own specialties and can do some truly amazing things to help you achieve the smile you want. I know that I'm grateful to have the experience and specialized skills to help my patients repair and enhance their smiles and their self-confidence. I also know that many other cosmetic dentists feel the same way.

When you need specialized care, you seek out a dentist with specialized knowledge. When you need cosmetic dentistry, then, it follows that you should seek out a cosmetic dentist, right? But even that might not be specific enough to ensure that you receive the best care possible and have the best options at your disposal. Your needs are unique, and it is important to take your time and find the dentist with the experience and knowledge needed to address each one.

Having a cosmetic dentist you can trust is incredibly important not only to your dental health but also to achieving your cosmetic dentistry goals! When you trust your cosmetic dentist, you are more likely to feel comfortable telling them about all of your dental desires. This is something that can only happen when you're comfortable enough with a dentist to work with them long-term and share the vision of your dream smile, which in turn helps them see the big picture. With that in mind, if you are planning on completing a smile transformation it is vitally important that you stick with the same dentist all the way through. Cosmetic dentists are like artists, and they craft a perfect plan for you and your smile.

Take the time to go in for a consult with the dentist you have in mind before making a final decision about who will handle your smile transformation. Ask your questions and be honest with yourself about whether they are someone you can see yourself working with to help your needs for both your smile and your mental health.

It can be difficult to narrow down who might be the best cosmetic dentist to enhance your smile. Because of this, I have outlined a few tips and questions you can use during your search.

Questions for Your Cosmetic Dentist

First of all, just knowing that you're looking specifically for a cosmetic dentist is half the battle. The other half of the battle comes down to comparing education, experience, and specialties to find the dentist who has the practical knowledge to help you. There are a few different things you should keep in mind when making a final decision. I wouldn't entirely discount a dentist's reviews, for example, as a large number of negative reviews (when compared to positive or neutral reviews) might say something about that dentist's ability to put their knowledge to work in a practical setting. As someone who has over 200 five-star reviews on Yelp, Google, and Facebook, and has been ranked #1 for three years straight, I can confidently say that user reviews and testimonials are only one part of the puzzle.

In order to find the dentist that will be best able to treat your needs, first, you must understand what you want to have done to your teeth. What are your goals? Once you have a goal in mind – even if it's a vague one – you can start to look at dentists around you and find the individuals who have the experience you need and those who don't. There is a wealth of information to be found online – utilize it to help find a particular cosmetic dentist's credentials. You want to look at their education, their experience, and their specialties. Make sure that the dentist you're interested in has experience with the kind of cosmetic dentistry that you are hoping to receive.

Something else to keep in mind is the amount of attention and detail given about the practice. Are there plenty of pictures of the dentist office? Do they offer the latest technology? For example, I offer things like iTero and Invisalign at my practice, and find that the most current technological advances are often to key creating perfect, healthy smiles.

If you aren't sure where to find a doctor's information or simply aren't sure what you might need to have done to your teeth in order to help meet your goals, don't be afraid to schedule consultations. Finding a dentist that is a good fit for you – one who can help you feel comfortable while also working to enhance your smile – is important, and sometimes you need an in-person visit to really understand whether or not this particular dentist is going to be able to help.

If you make the decision to go in for a consultation, make sure to write down any questions you might have for the dentist regarding your teeth as well as their experience. It's okay to ask someone if they've done the kind of work you're facing.

- Will you be their first patient, or have they done this procedure before?
- What exactly will they be doing to your teeth – which procedures will be performed?
- Do they feel comfortable performing this kind of work?

The above questions are just a start to help you think of information you'd like to have. As I mentioned earlier, many people simply look at a dentist's title and think that it's good enough. They don't dig into their backgrounds and are scared to ask questions. You don't have to be that person! Look at someone's professional history. Do they belong to any professional associations? What are their academic credentials? Have they been recognized for their work? It is important for my patients, and potential patients to know that I have been recognized for work that I've done and received an education at a world-renowned dental college. It helps them rest assured that I know what I'm doing and am comfortable working on their teeth.

A few more things to can keep in mind when looking for a dentist – and a few that might even help if you end up scheduling a consultation are:

- Is cosmetic dentistry their focus?
- Do they have any before and after pictures that showcase their results?
- What level of postgraduate education do they have in dental education?
- Are there reviews online that you can read to help get a better "feel" for a dentist's bedside manner and overall results?
- Do you feel comfortable with them?
- What treatment options can they offer you?

Considering treatment options is a particularly important thing to keep in mind. Inquire about the levels of treatment options the dentist can offer you. It's likely that there is an "ideal" option in their mind as well as other viable options that might not seem as optimal for various reasons. These options are important to have because, ultimately, we're talking about your teeth and your smile. You should be the person to make the final call regarding what kind of work you wish to pursue.

In addition to ensuring your potential cosmetic dentist has the education you need, make sure they have the experience to help guarantee good results, too. This might also be a personal preference of sorts. It all comes down to comfort. If you're comfortable with the level of experience that a dentist has, then there's no problem. It's still a good idea to look for experienced cosmetic dentists in your area, however, as they are the most equipped to adapt their treatment options should unexpected complications arise.

Finally, make sure that you ask for information about sedation methods the clinic offers to ensure that you receive the care that is right for you. Not every clinic will offer the same types of sedation. This is important to keep in mind if you know that you need help to make it through an appointment or will be receiving procedures that will result in your sedation in some way, shape, or form. Also, ask about aftercare processes and what you can expect once the treatment is completed.

It is a good idea to ask these questions before you go in for a specific treatment so that you have a good understanding of what to expect and what can be done to make you most comfortable. Don't hesitate to be honest with the staff and ask them for their advice regarding what kind of sedation methods might work best for you.

Choosing to enhance your smile can enrich your life and lead to more happiness. This process should be an exciting journey for you, one that can open up your life to new and happy opportunities. But, as shown above, this choice does not lead to the same path for everyone. And, is best done when you have complete trust in the cosmetic dentist you have chosen to address the needs of your smile. To best approach your journey in enhancing your smile, be sure to research beyond the information provided here and speak with a professional cosmetic dentist. My goal is to make you proud of your smile in every way, and together, I am sure we can make that happen.

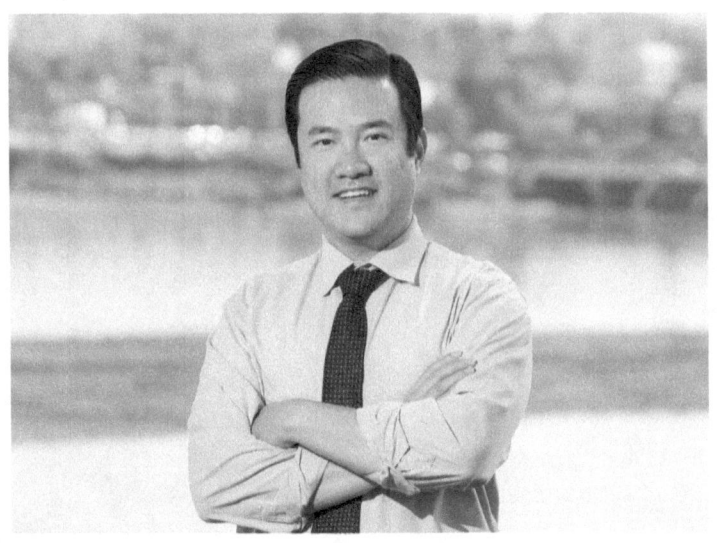

Dr. Mark K Nguyen DDS is an acclaimed cosmetic dentist located in the Costa Mesa, California, region. He offers his patient award-winning cosmetic dental work including dental implants, veneers, professional teeth whitening, and Invisalign clear aligners, among other services. His work has been detailed and featured in Orange Coast Magazine and VoyageLA, and he works tirelessly to give his patients the smile of their dreams. He currently practices at OC Healthy Smiles with a skilled team of colleagues and office staff.